Mediterranean Sweet Temptations

50 Delicious & Healthy Sweet Recipes for Your Mediterranean Diet

Alex Brawn

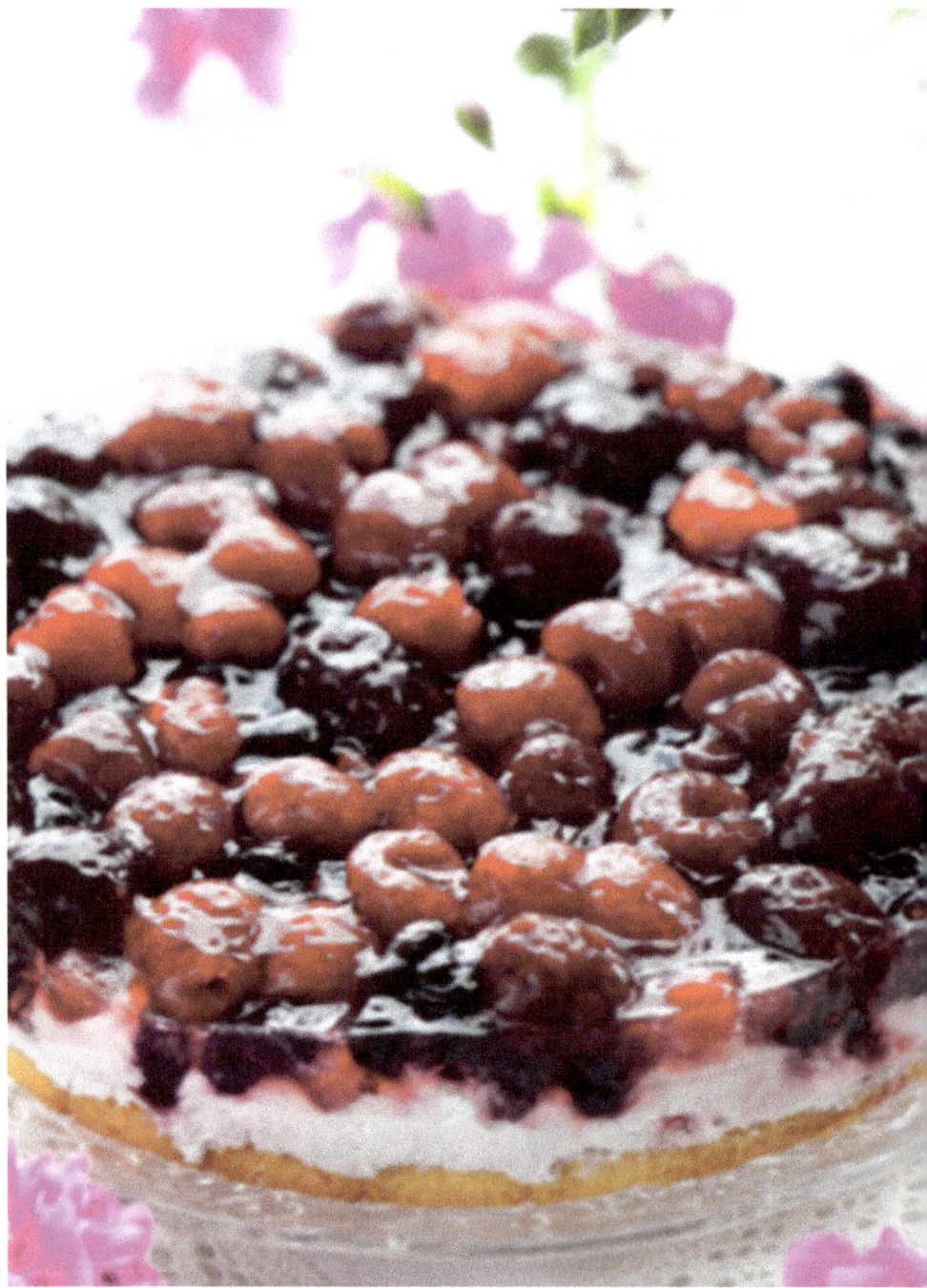

By reading this document, the reader agrees that under no circumstances is the author responsible for any losses, direct or indirect, which are incurred as a result of the use of information contained within this document, including, but not limited to, — errors, omissions, or inaccuracies.

Table of Contents

Classic apple crumble

The classic apple crumble is a homely Mediterranean fruit recipe, simple and delicious for breakfast.

Ingredients

- 100g of plain flour
- 150g golden caster sugar
- 1 lemon
- 50g of unsalted butter
- 1.5kg of mixed apples

Directions

- Preheat your oven to 400°F.
- Peel and core the apples.
- Place in a saucepan over medium heat with sugar and some gratings of lemon zest.
- Cook for 5 minutes with the lid on.
- Lower the heat and let cool.
- Place butter in a mixing bowl with flour.
- Rub together with your fingertips until it resembles breadcrumbs and add the remaining sugar.
- Transfer the apples to a baking dish.

- Sprinkle over the crumble topping.
- Bake for 25 to 30 minutes.
- Serve and enjoy with vanilla.

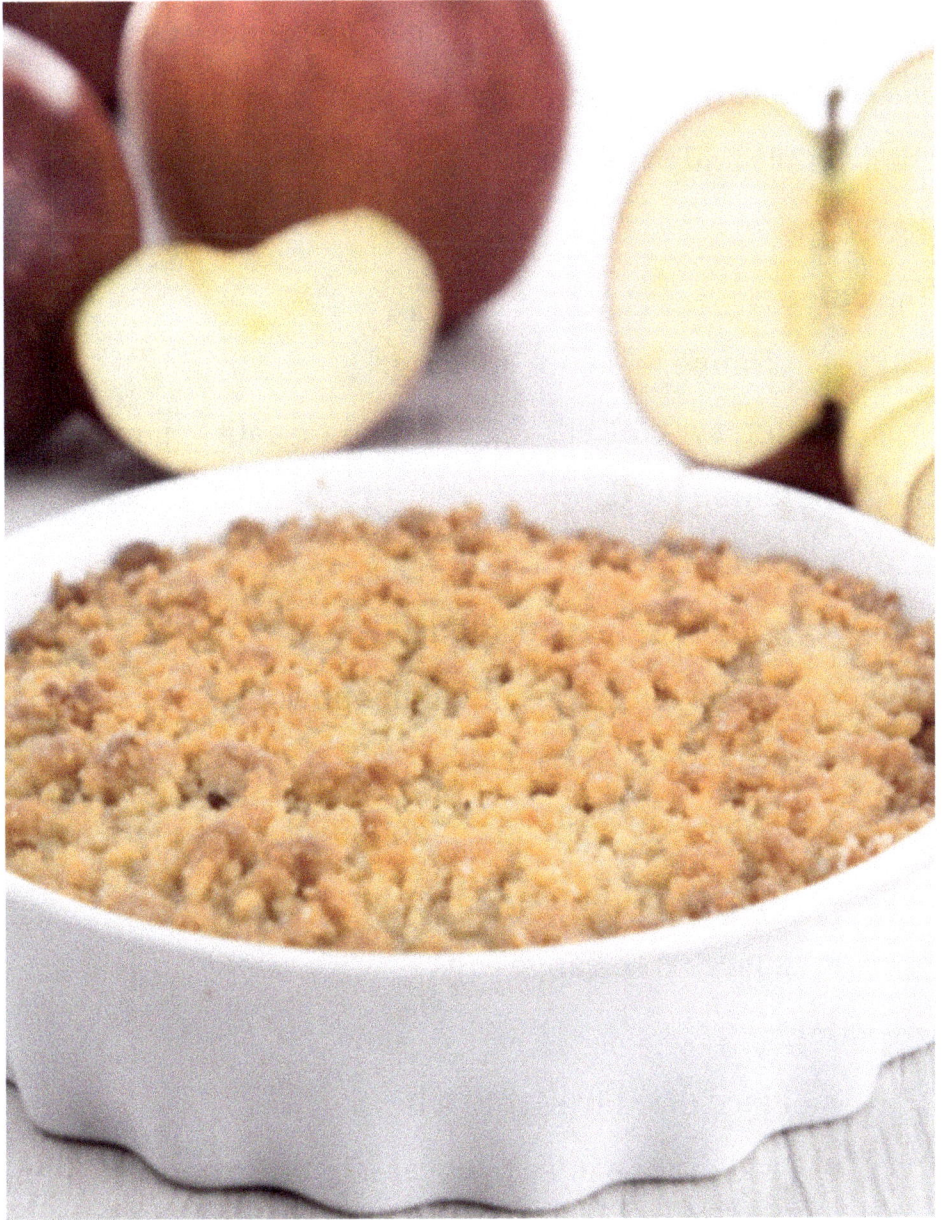

Crumbliest scones

Following these procedures for making scones can yield better of this meal than a store bought scones. They are quiet simple and ease to make, tasty when still fresh from the oven.

Ingredients

- Orange juice, for soaking
- Jersey clotted cream, good-quality jam or lemon curd
- 4 tablespoons of milk
- 500g of self-rising flour
- 2 level teaspoons of baking powder
- 150g of dried fruit
- 2 heaped teaspoons of golden caster sugar
- 150g of cold unsalted butter
- 2 large free-range eggs

Directions

- Place dried fruit into a bowl.
- Add orange juice to cover let stay for hours.
- Preheat your oven to 400°F.

- Combine the butter, flour, sugar, baking powder, and a good pinch of sea salt ina mixing bowl.
- Break and rub the butter with your fingers.
- Make a well in the middle of the dough.
- Add eggs and milk.
- Stir up with a spatula.
- Drain soaked fruit, add to the mixture.
- Add a tiny splash of milk.
- Sprinkle over some flour, cover the bowl with Clingfilm, keep in the fridge briefly.
- Roll the dough out on a lightly floured surface until it's about 3cm thick.
- Cut out circles from the dough and place them upside down on a baking sheet.
- Brush the top of each scone with the extra milk.
- Bake in the oven for 15 minutes.
- Serve and enjoy with clotted cream.

Apple and walnut risotto with gorgonzola

Ingredients

- Freshly ground black pepper
- 1 basic risotto recipe
- 1 handful of walnuts
- 75g of soft goat's cheese, crumbled
- 700ml of organic vegetable
- Extra virgin olive oil
- 50g of butter
- 1 small handful of Parmesan cheese
- 1 small bunch of fresh marjoram
- Sea salt
- 175g of gorgonzola cheese, diced
- 2 crunchy eating apples

Directions

- Place a large saucepan on a medium to high heat.
- Pour in half the stock, then the risotto base.
- Bring to the boil, stirring all the time, lower the heat, let simmer until almost all the stock has been absorbed.

- Add the rest of the stock, bit by bit until the rice is cooked.
- Turn off the heat, beat in the butter together with the Parmesan, goat's cheese, chopped apple, gorgonzola, and marjoram.
- Taste, and adjust the seasoning.
- Let the risotto rest briefly, covered with a lid.
- Heat the walnuts in a pan.
- Serve and enjoy with a sprinkle of the walnuts and drizzle with a little extra virgin olive oil.

Apple and cranberry sauce

Ingredients

- 1 stick of cinnamon
- 500g of cranberries
- 150g of golden caster sugar
- 2 bramley apples

Directions

- Place all the ingredients in a wide saucepan with a splash of water.
- Place the pan on heat and bring to the boil.
- Simmer gently until the cranberries have burst and the apple are soft.
- Boil down until the mixture thickens slightly.
- Remove, let cool.
- Serve and enjoy.

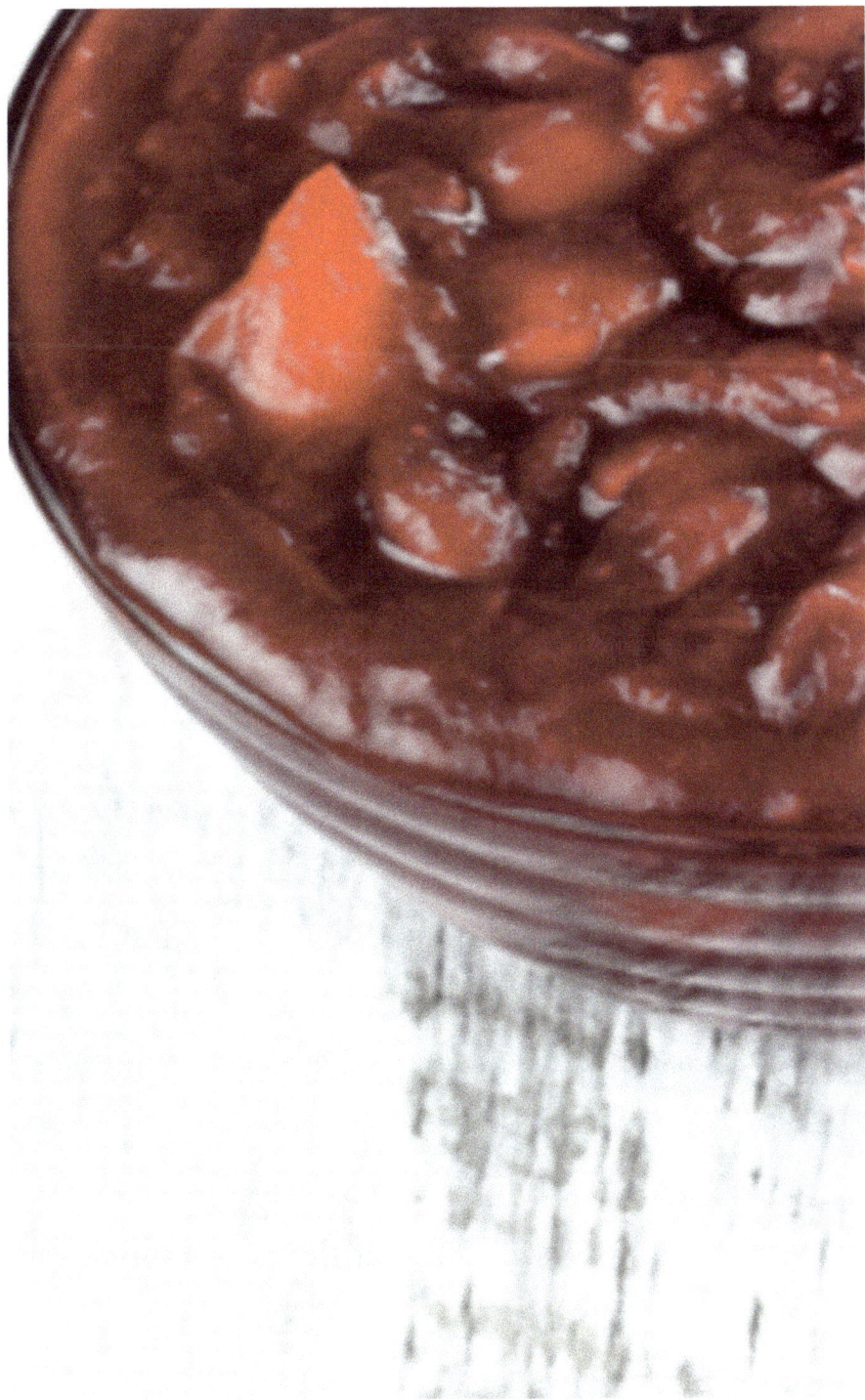

Summer crunch salad with walnuts and gorgonzola

Ingredients

- 200g of gorgonzola cheese
- 1 lemon
- Extra virgin olive oil
- 2 bulbs fennel, thinly sliced
- 3 large handfuls fresh peas
- 2 handfuls walnut halves
- 2 small red apples

Directions

- Squeeze the lemon through your fingers into a mixing bowl, make sure to catch any pips.
- Add 3 times as much olive oil to the lemon juice.
- Season with sea salt and freshly ground black pepper. Whisk.
- Core and thinly slice each apple.
- Then, toss with the fennel and walnuts in the dressing.
- Divide between smaller dishes.

- Crumble the Gorgonzola over the top of each.
- Serve and enjoy.

Apple and celeriac soup

Ingredients

- A few sage leaves
- A few sprigs of thyme
- 4 tablespoons of olive oil
- 4 apples
- 2 liters of vegetable stock
- 2 onions
- Toasted hazelnuts
- 200ml of crème fraiche
- 1 celery stalk
- 1 celeriac

Directions

- Heat half of the olive oil in a large pan.
- Cook slice onions with chopped celery over a medium heat for 10 minutes, or until soft.
- Chop the celeriac, core and quarter the apples, add to the pan with thyme leaves, let cook for 3 minutes.

- Add the stock, season, over low heat let simmer for 30 minutes until the celeriac is tender.
- Remove from heat, blend until smooth. Stir in half the crème fraiche.
- Heat the remaining oil in a pan and fry the sage leaves until crispy.
- Spoon the soup into bowls, topping with the remaining crème fraiche.
- Drizzle with extra virgin olive oil and sprinkle with the crispy sage leaves and hazelnuts.
- Enjoy.

Waldorf salad

Ingredients

- 2 crisp eating apples
- 150g of grapes
- 6 sprigs of fresh tarragon
- 250ml of fat-free natural yoghurt
- 2 sticks of celery
- 1 lemon
- Olive oil
- 1 teaspoon of English mustard
- 60g of shelled walnuts
- 1 cos, or Romaine lettuce

Directions

- Preheat your oven ready to 350°F.
- Place the grapes on a baking tray, finely grate over the zest from ½ the lemon, and drizzle with a little oil.
- Season with sea salt and black pepper.
- Then, place in the hot oven for 15 minutes.
- Add the walnuts, let roast for more 10 minutes.

- Place the mustard with yoghurt into a dish, whisk.
- Add the chopped tarragon leaves and squeeze in the lemon juice, mix, then season to taste.
- Place chopped celery and sliced apples, lettuce, grapes into a large bowl.
- Drizzle over the yoghurt dressing and toss well.
- Place onto a platter, roughly chop and sprinkle over the walnuts.
- Serve and enjoy.

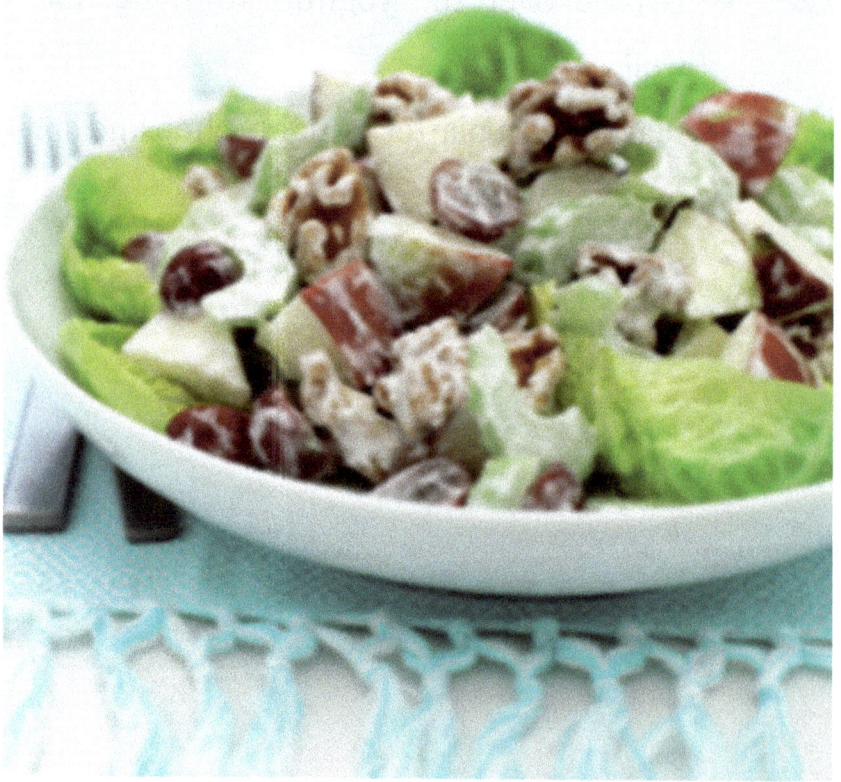

Parsnips and shell nut tart tatin

Ingredients

- 1 tablespoon Dijon mustard
- ½ bramley apple
- 20g of goose fat
- ½ tablespoon of balsamic vinegar
- 50g of unsalted butter
- ½ tablespoon of runny honey
- 2 parsnips
- 100g of ready-to-cook shell nuts
- 7 sprigs of thyme
- 320g if ready-rolled puff pastry
- ½ tablespoon of dark brown sugar
- 3 shallots
- 1 tablespoon of balsamic vinegar
- 200g of shallots
- 50g of dates
- ½ tablespoon of olive oil

Directions

- Preheat the oven to 400°F.

- Heat olive oil in a medium pan over a medium-low heat.
- Add the shallots, let cook for 5 minutes, until tender.
- Stir in the mustard together with the balsamic, dates, honey, sugar, and water.
- Season, and lower the heat, let cook for 15 minutes, stirring occasionally,
- Remove, let cool.
- Heat the goose fat and butter in an ovenproof frying pan over a medium-low heat.
- Then, add the parsnips together with the shallots, cut-side down, let cook until it begins to caramelize.
- Add the shell nuts with thyme sprigs, season, let cook for 5 minutes.
- Remove from the heat and top with half of the shallot compote.
- Roll out the pastry and trim it so it's slightly bigger than the pan.
- Remove the pan from the heat and roll the pastry over the top.

- Let bake for 30 minutes, until the pastry is golden.
- Simmer the apple with water in a small pan over a medium heat for 10 minutes.
- Season and stir in the balsamic.
- Serve and enjoy hot with the apple balsamic sauce on the side.

Cheat's cranberry sauce

Ingredients

- 1 x 250g jar of cranberry sauce
- 1 eating apple
- 1 cinnamon stick
- 1 fresh bay leaf
- 1 knob of unsalted butter

Directions

- Place a pan on a medium heat with the butter, cinnamon, and bay.
- Let cook briefly for 40 seconds, or until the cinnamon starts to catch and burn.
- Stir in the cubes of apple and a swig of water, shake to coat in the butter.
- Leave to soften for a couple of minutes.
- Pour in the cranberry sauce, let warm through.
- Serve and enjoy.

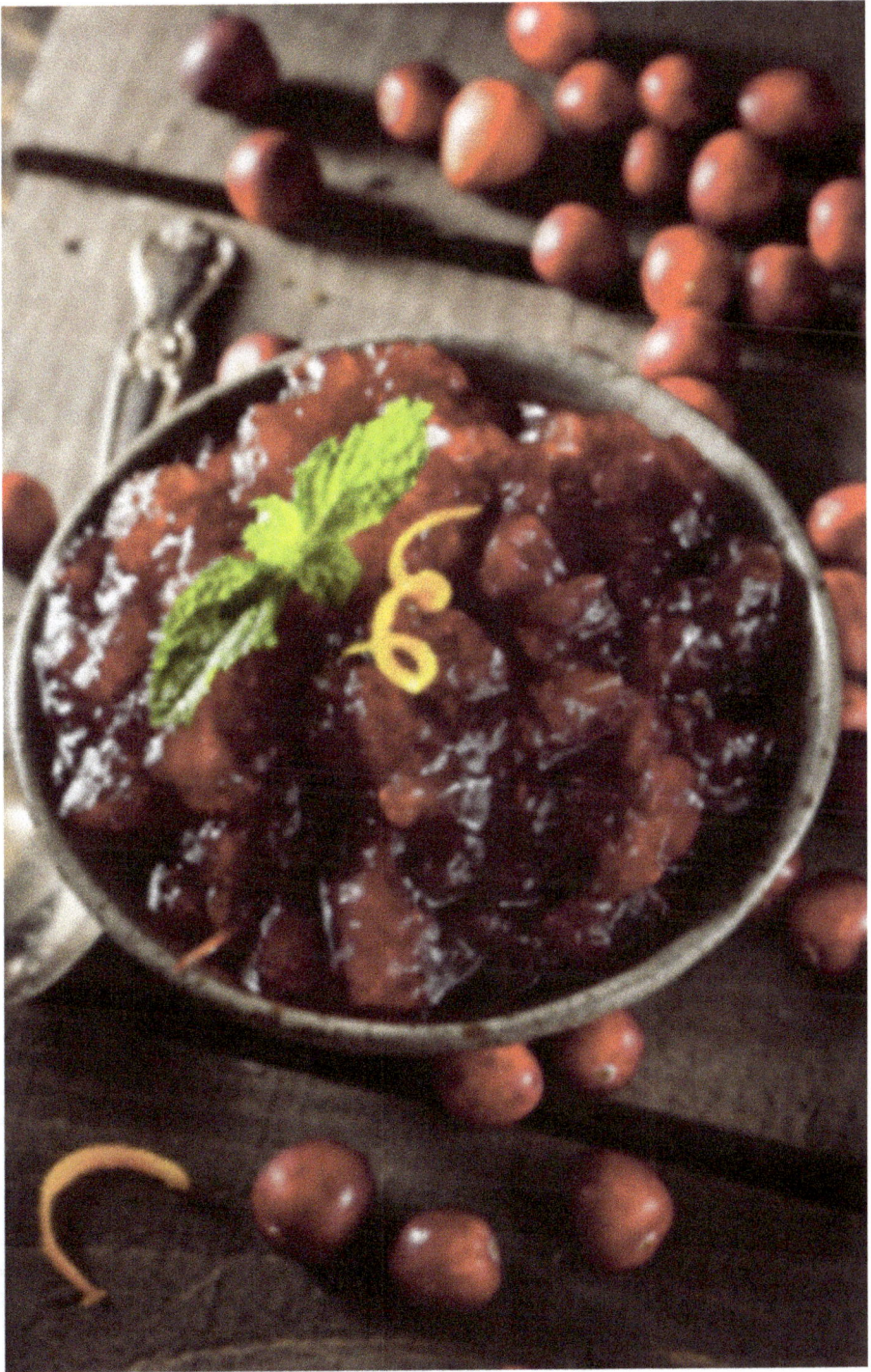

Grapefruit, carrots, and apple juice

Ingredients

- ½ of a grapefruit
- 1 apple
- 3 medium carrots

Directions

- Peel the grapefruit, and quarter the apple.
- Push the grapefruit with the carrots and apple through a juicer, straight into a glass.
- Stir well.
- Enjoy.

Blue cheese and apple burger

Ingredients

- Mustard
- 750g of minced chuck steak
- 6 burger buns
- 1 soft round lettuce
- Olive oil
- 120g of blue cheese
- 1 punnet of cress
- 2 Brae burn

Directions

- Divide the mince into 4 portions and work each ball in your hands for a few minutes to melt the fat.
- Mold them into a relatively smooth, round patty. Make sure they are bigger than the burns.
- Place them on a tray cover with Clingfilm, let chill in the fridge.
- Preheat your grill to high.

- Place a large non-stick frying pan over a medium heat and add a drizzle of oil to the pan.
- Let fry the burgers for 4 minutes on each side.
- Seasoning the patties with black pepper as you cook them.
- Halve and toast the buns under the grill, then line them up on a board ready to go.
- When the burgers are cooked, top each with the blue cheese, place under the grill for a couple of minutes until oozy.
- Now build your burgers. First layer the salad leaves and apple onto the buns, then drizzle of mustard.
- Place the burgers on, topping with the cress.
- Enjoy your delicious.

Fried cox apples with cinnamon sugar

Ingredients

- 1 teaspoon of ground cinnamon
- 250g of unsalted butter
- 4 tablespoons of caster sugar
- 4 Cox orange pippin apple
- Apple juice
- 1 lemon

Directions

- Begin by clarifying the butter by boiling in a small pan.
- Strain into a container through a sieve lined with a coffee filter.
- Peel, core and slice each apple into 8, then sprinkle over a little lemon juice to prevent the slices from browning.
- Heat some clarified butter in a non-stick frying pan.
- Add the apple pieces in one layer.
- Let cook until the undersides are nicely tanned.

- Combine the sugar together with the cinnamon, turn over the apple slices and sprinkle with the cinnamon sugar.
- Lift the apples into a dish.
- Pour a splash of the apple juice in the pan.
- Serve and enjoy.

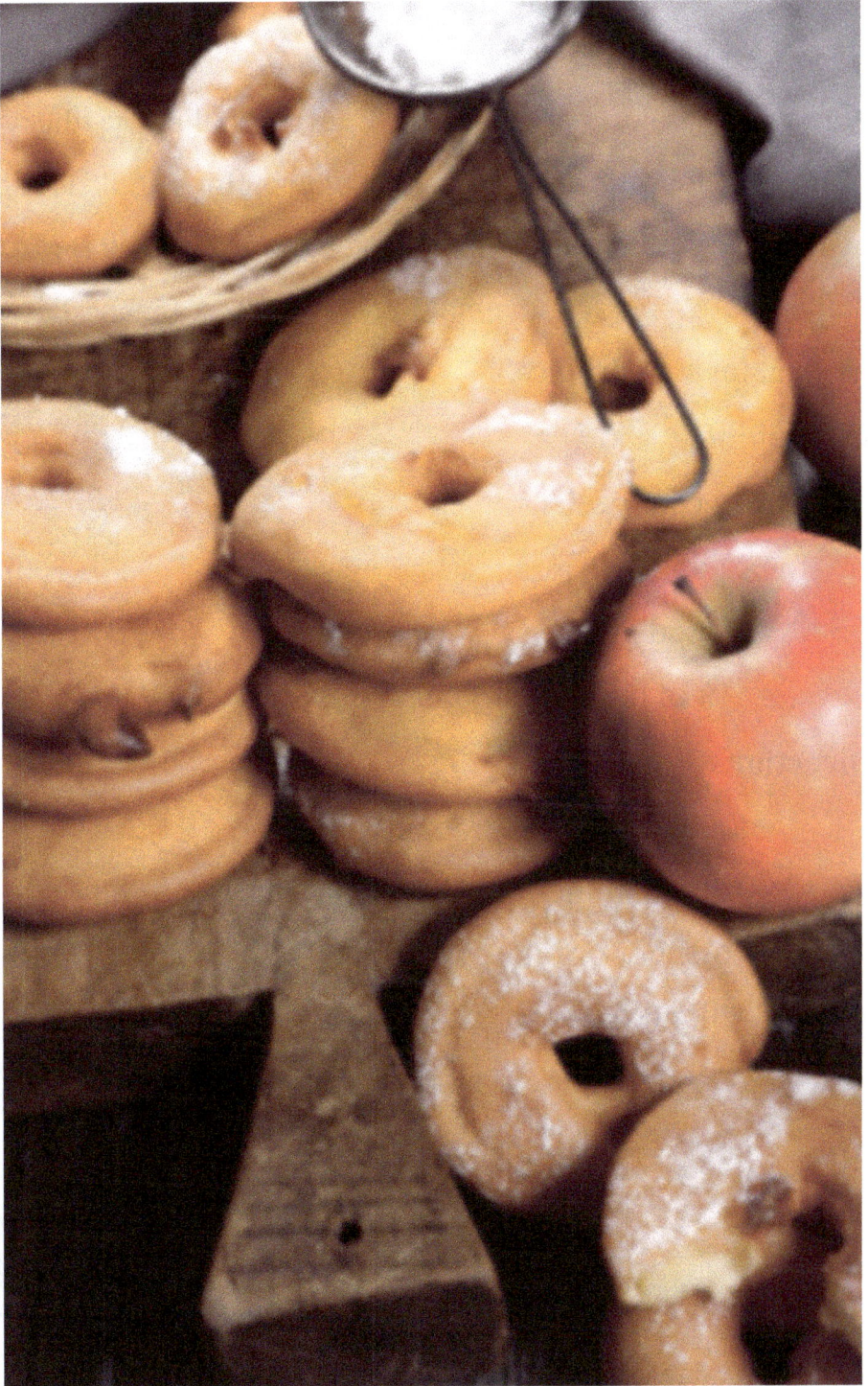

Celery juice

The celery juice is an excellent source of dietary fiber significant for calorie weight loss plans. More so, it is a tasty and a refreshing with a rejuvenating property for a daily diet. A person cannot love Mediterranean diet without loving this juice.

Ingredients

- 2 celery sticks
- 1 apple
- ¼ od ginger
- ¼ of lime or lemon

Directions

- Clean all the ingredients.
- Place all ingredients except lime or lemon in a blender or juicer
- Blend thoroughly.
- Squeeze lemon over the juice
- Serve and enjoy chilled.

Apple ginger juice

Ingredients

- 3 apples
- ½ piece of ginger
- ½ lemon
- ½ cup of water

Directions

- Clean and chop the apples.
- Combine apple, ginger and the water in the juicer.
- Squeeze the lemon in.
- Blend until smooth puree.
- Strain and sieve the juice.
- Serve and enjoy immediately.

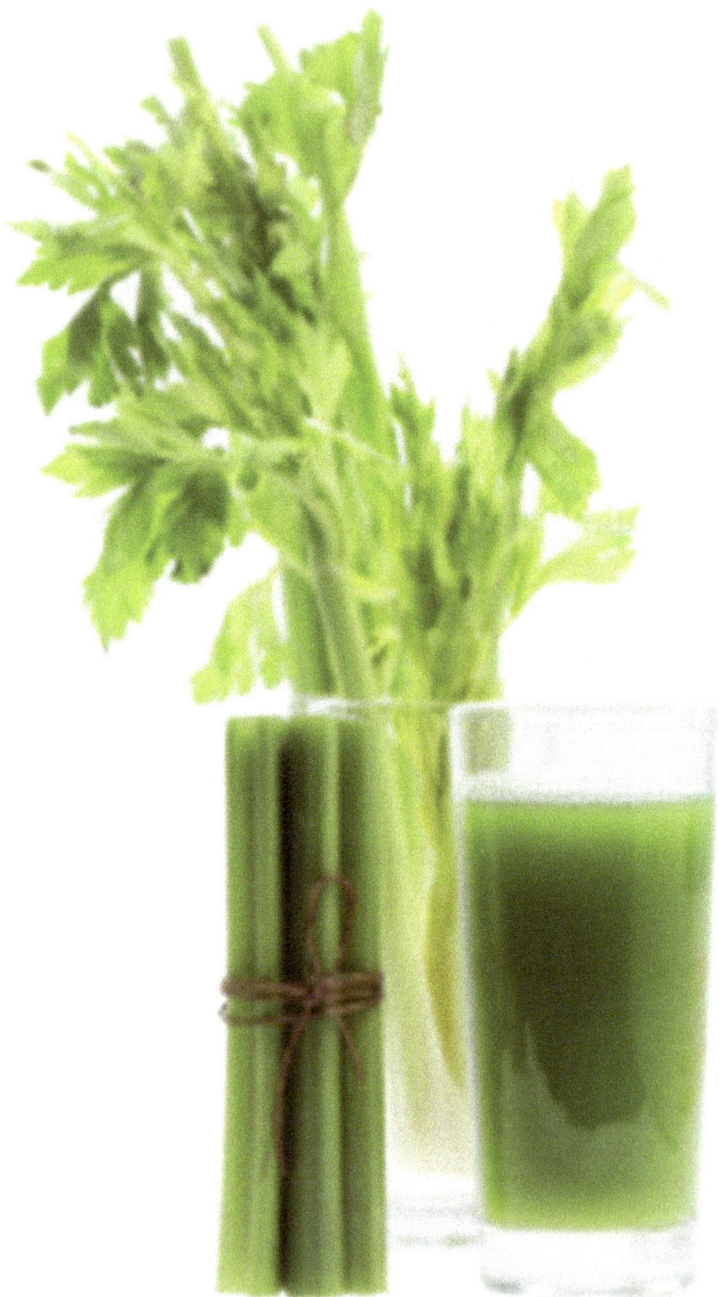

Grape juice

This is an easy Mediterranean Sea diet juice to make even if one does not have a blender. It contains several vitamins mainly vitamins C, A, K, and B-complex which is paramount in protecting the body against viral and fungal infections.

Ingredients

- 2 cups of sweet ripe black grapes
- ½ lemon
- 1 cup of water
- 8 ice cubes.

Directions

- Clean and place the grapes in a blender.
- Add the water.
- Run the blender until smooth.
- Strain and sieve, and then squeeze the lemon over.
- Adjust the thickness with more water.
- Serve and enjoy chilled or at room temperature.

Strawberry raspberry smoothie

Ingredients

- ½ cup of raspberries
- ½ cup of frozen strawberries
- ½ of banana
- ¼ cup of plain yogurt
- ½ of almond milk
- ½ teaspoon of chia seeds
- ½ tablespoon of honey

Directions

- Pour almond milk together with the yogurt in a blender.
- Then, add the raspberries, banana, chia seeds, honey, and strawberries.
- Run the blender until smooth.
- Serve and enjoy.

17. Pomegranate juice

Ingredients

- 1 cup of fresh pomegranate seeds
- ½ cup of water

Directions

- Cut and remove the pomegranate crown, and make shallow cuts on the skin, make sure to deseed.
- Place 1 cup of pomegranate seeds in a blender.
- Add the water.
- Pulse to break the seeds a little.
- Strain and sieve.
- Serve and enjoy.

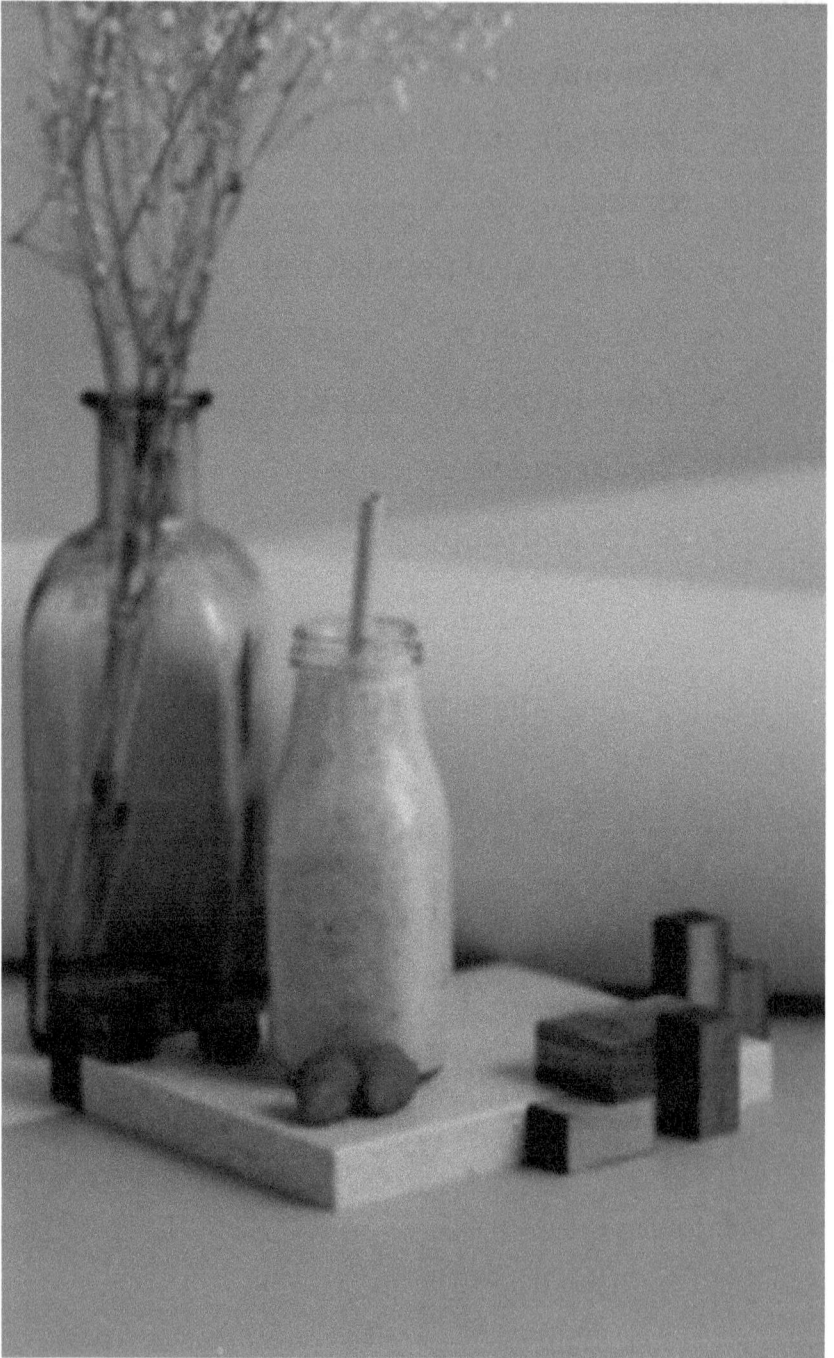

Strawberry juice

Ingredients

- 2 cups of ripe strawberries
- 1 tablespoon of honey
- 1 cup of cold water
- 2 ice cubes
- 1 halves strawberry

Directions

- Combine the strawberries together with the honey in a blender.
- Blend until smooth puree.
- Add water, blend briefly.
- Serve with ice cubes and halved strawberries on the rim of the serving glasses.

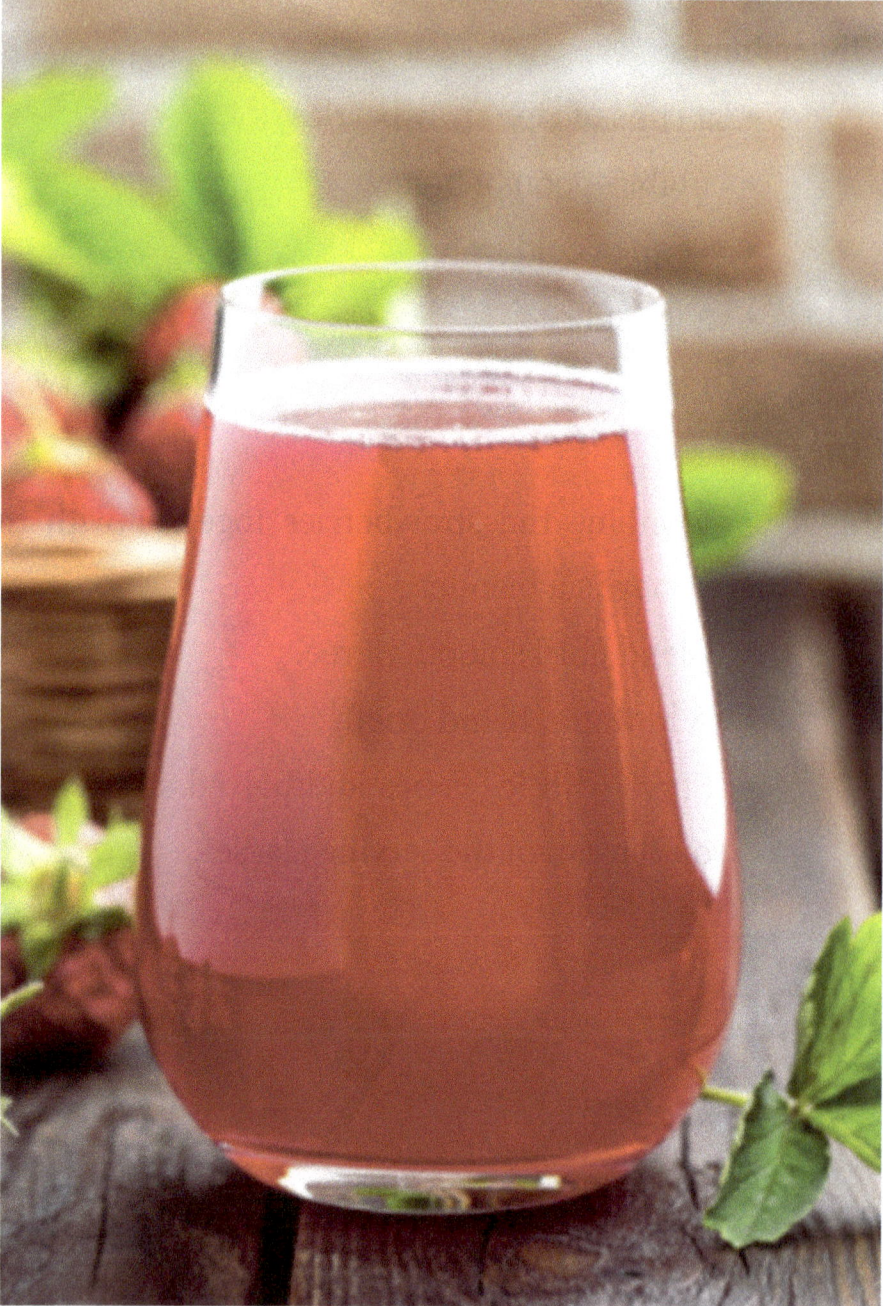

Orange pineapple juice

This Mediterranean Sea diet juice is largely an orange juice with little taste of pineapple. The orange pineapple juice is a tasty and delicious recipe, but its health and nutrition benefits supersedes its taste.

Ingredients

- 4 oranges
- 1 pinch of ground black pepper
- 1 cup of water
- Salt
- 2 cups of chopped ripe pineapples
- Honey

Directions

- Cut and halve the oranges.
- Squeeze the juice with a juicer.
- Place pineapples, honey, sugar, salt, and ground black pepper in a blender.
- Blend until smooth puree.
- Strain, then add the orange juice, mix.
- Serve and enjoy.

Pineapple juice

Ingredients

- 1/2 ripe pineapple
- ½ cup of water
- 6 ice cubes
- Honey

Directions

- place chopped pineapple and water in a blender.
- Process until smooth puree without chunks.
- Strain properly.
- Add ice cubes and stir well.
- Taste and adjust sweetness accordingly.
- Serve and enjoy.

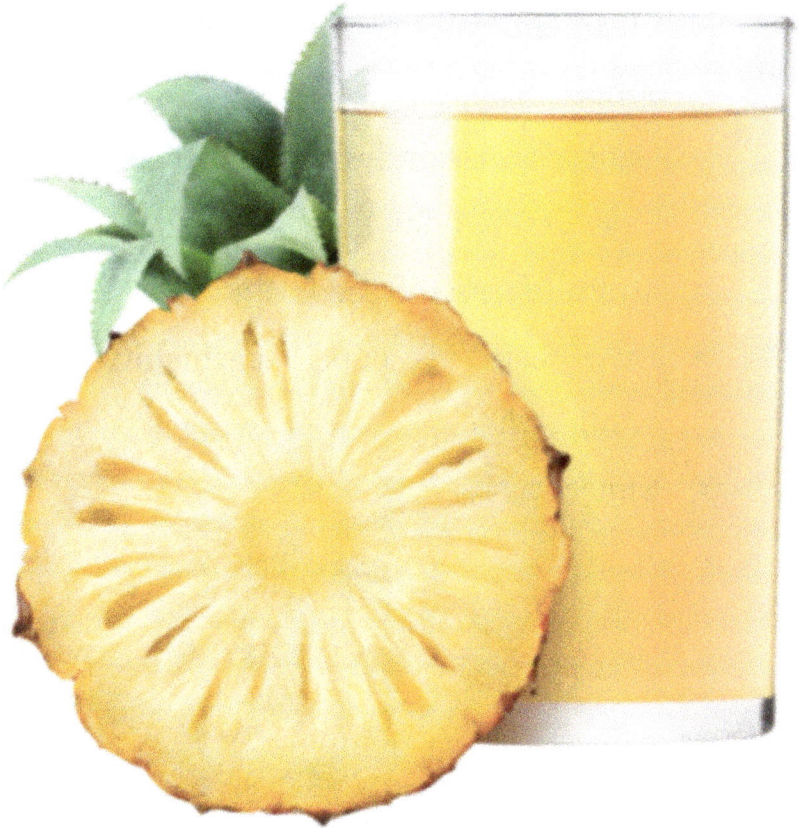

Orange juice

Ingredients

- 3 fresh oranges
- Ice cubes

Directions

- Clean and roll the oranges on a flat surface to soften.
- Cut crosswise and place in a juicer.
- Squeeze the juice.
- Strain to trap the seeds.
- Serve with ice cubes, garnishing with the orange wheel.
- Enjoy.

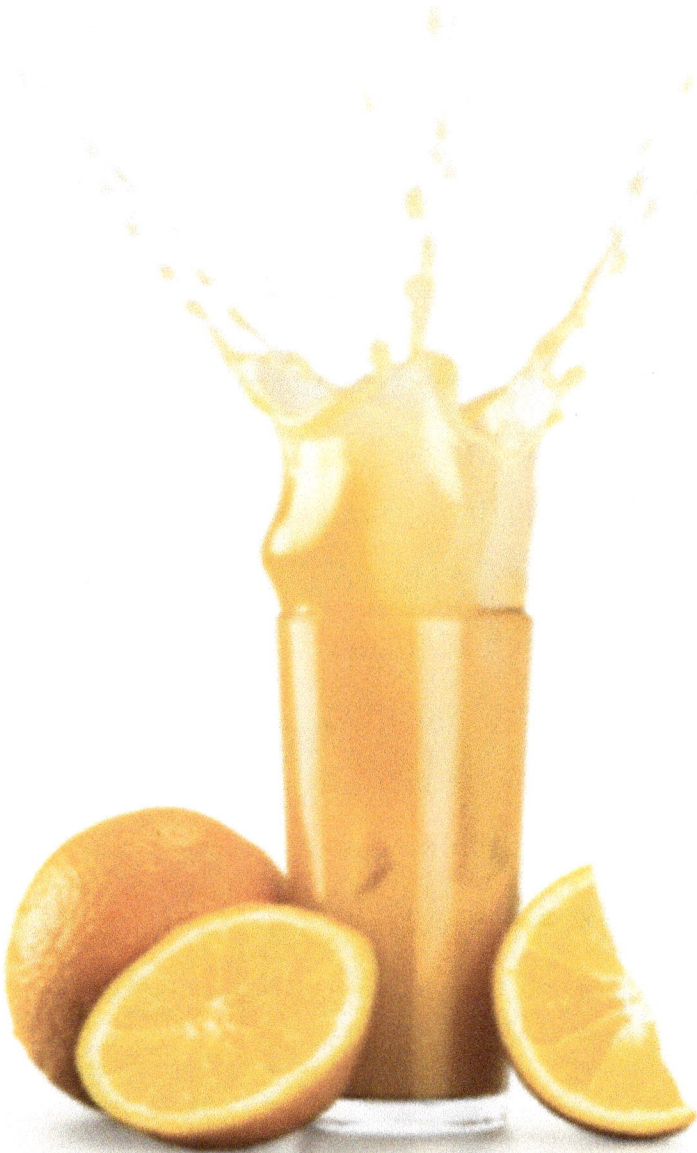

Apple orange juice

Ingredients

- 1 sweet apple
- 2 oranges
- ¾ cup of water
- 2 teaspoons of honey

Directions

- Chop and prepare the oranges, remove the skin and seeds.
- Place in a juicer, and squeeze out the juice.
- Add water, chopped apples, and juice from the oranges in a blender.
- Blend until smooth puree.
- Strain.
- Then, add honey, mix.
- Serve and enjoy.

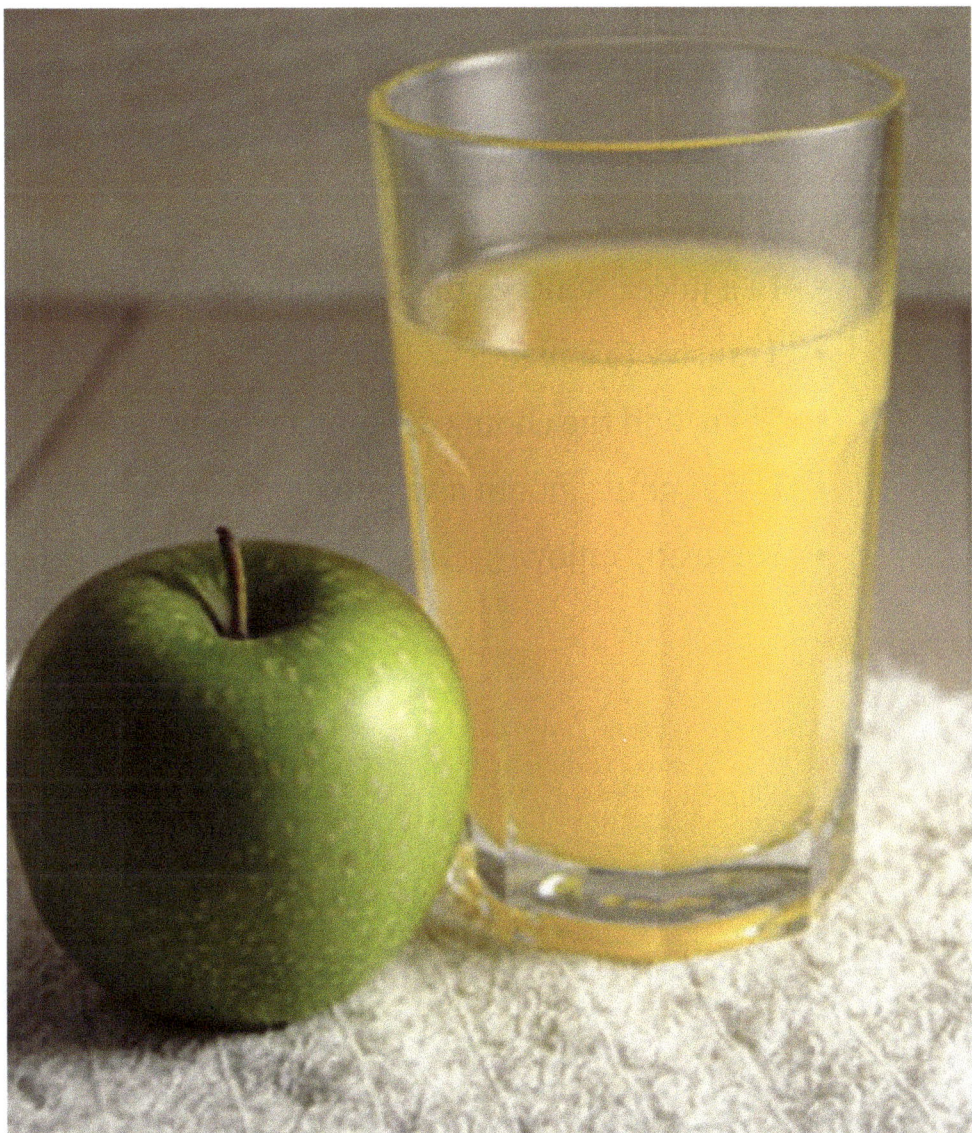

Banana orange juice

Ingredients

- 2 oranges
- 6 ice cubes
- 1 medium banana

Directions

- In a juicer, squeeze the lemon juice.
- Transfer to a blender.
- Then, add the chopped banana with ice cubes.
- Blend until smooth and puree.
- Serve and enjoy.

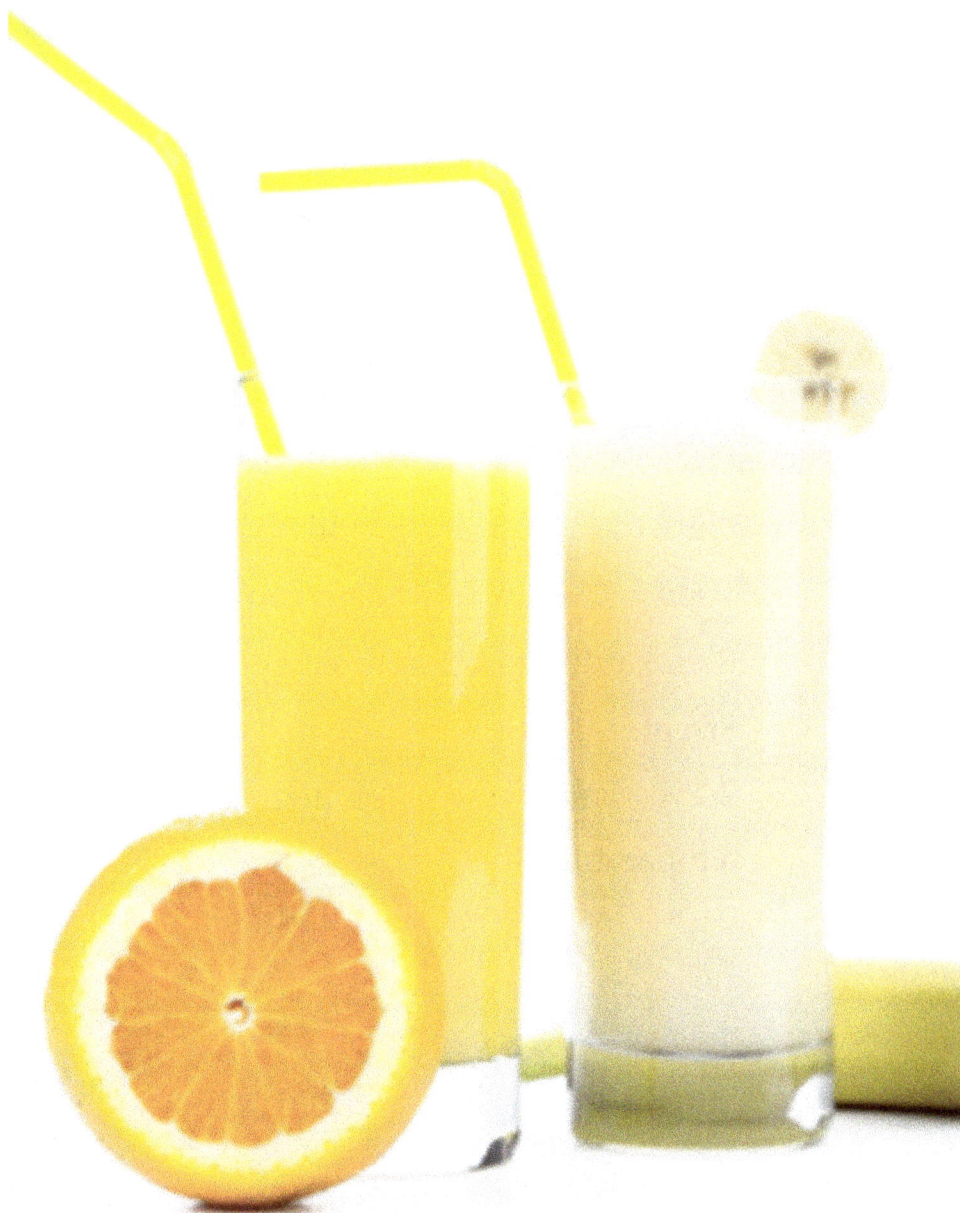

Fresh spinach juice

Ingredients

- 2 cups of chopped spinach
- 1 stalk of celery
- Juice from ½ lemon
- ¾ cup of water
- 1 apple

Ingredients

- Place the apple, celery, and water in a blender.
- Then, add the spinach and lemon juice.
- Blend until smooth without chunks.
- Strain.
- Serve and enjoy chilled or at room temperature.

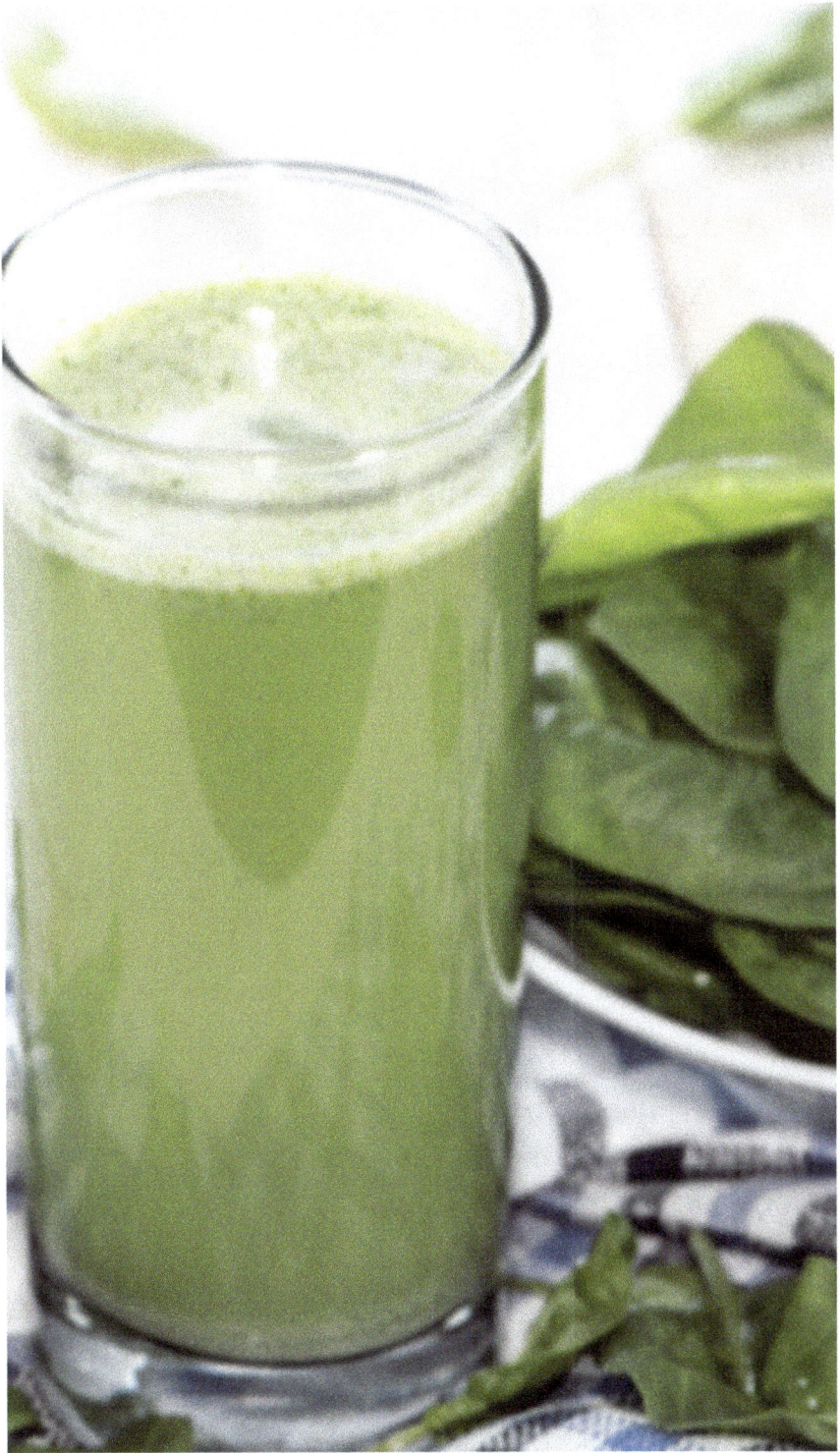

Kiwi juice

Ingredients

- 1 celery stalk
- Apple
- Kiwifruit

Directions

- Clean and slice the apple and kiwifruit.
- Place the slices of apples and kiwifruit with celery stalk in a juicer.
- Process using an omega masticating juicer.
- Serve and enjoy.

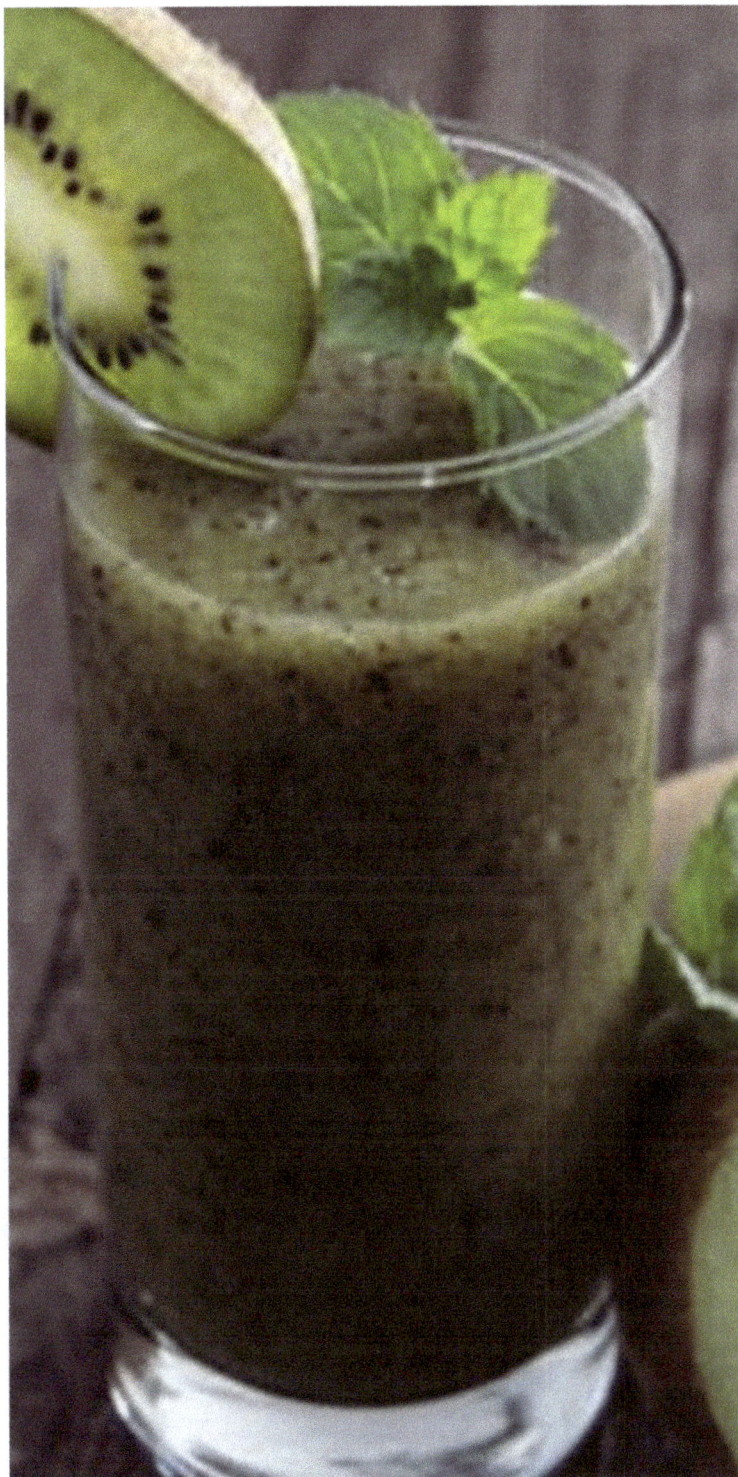

Papaya juice

Ingredients

- 2 teaspoons of lemon juice
- ½ medium size papaya
- ½ cup of fresh pineapple juice
- 2 teaspoons of honey
- 1/8 teaspoon of black pepper powder
- Salt
- Water

Directions

- Place the papaya, pineapple juice, black pepper powder, lemon juice, honey, salt, and water in a blender.
- Blend until smooth puree.
- Check and adjust the consistency with pineapple juice, blend briefly.
- Taste, and adjust the sweetness with honey or lemon juice, making it tangy.
- Serve and enjoy chilled.

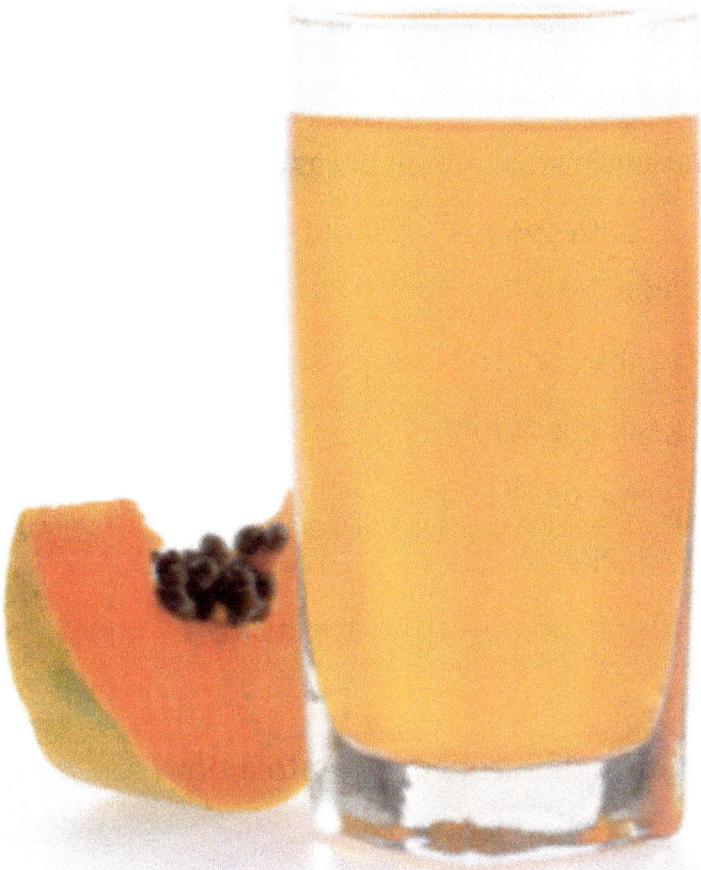

Sweetheart slaw with passion fruit dressing

Ingredients

- 1 carrot
- 1 sweetheart cabbage
- 1 large orange
- 3 large spears of asparagus
- 2 tablespoons of cold-pressed extra virgin olive oil
- 1 tablespoon of poppy seeds
- 3 spring onions
- 3 ripe passionfruit
- 2 sticks of celery
- 1 large green eating apple

Directions

- Grate the orange zest into a bowl and squeeze in all the juice.
- Halve the passion fruit and scrape in the pulp, then add the olive oil, mix together.
- Place shredded cabbage, asparagus, spring onions, apple, and carrot into a large bowl.

- Pour over the dressing, mix, season to taste.
- Serve and enjoy immediately.

Ultimate flapjacks

This Mediterranean Sea diet fruit recipe is a daily winner in most restaurants because of its taste and delicacy.

Ingredients

- 350g of rolled porridge oats
- 250g of soft light brown sugar
- 4 tablespoons of runny honey
- 250g of unsalted butter
- 100g of mixed nuts
- 150g of mixed dried fruit
- 1 pinch of sea salt

Directions

- Preheat your oven to 300°F.
- Grease, line a rectangular cake tin ready.
- Combine the butter, sugar, honey and salt in a medium pan over a low heat.
- Let the butter melt, stirring occasionally.
- Stir in the nuts and dried fruits in the pan along with the oats.
- Transfer the mixture to the prepared tin, smoothing it out into an even layer.

- Bake in the oven for 40 minutes.
- let cool completely, then cut into squares.
- Serve and enjoy.

Orange polenta cake

Ingredients

- 100g of fine polenta
- 200g of ground almonds
- 250g of runny honey
- 3 large free-range eggs
- 10 regular oranges

Directions

- Preheat your oven to 325°F.
- Rub a cake tin with olive oil, then line the base with greaseproof paper oiled.
- Squeeze the juice of 3 oranges into a pan.
- Add 100g of honey and simmer until thickened.
- Lower heat, remove from the heat.
- Whisk olive oil with the remaining 150g of honey for 2 minutes.
- Beat in the eggs for 2 minutes, as you grate and add the zest of 3 oranges.
- Stop the mixer, then fold in the ground almonds, polenta, and the juice of 2 oranges.

- Pour into the tin let bake for 50 minutes.
- Let cool for 10 minutes in the tin.
- Peel and slice the remaining oranges.
- Drizzle with syrup over everything before tucking in.
- Serve and enjoy.

Buddy's one cup pancakes

These pan cakes are very soft and fluffy. No weighing scales used but rather cups to improve its delicacy for a wonderful breakfast.

Ingredients

- Seasonal berries
- Runny honey or maple syrup
- 1 cup of semi-skimmed milk
- Natural yoghurt
- 1 large free-range egg
- Unsalted butter or olive oil, for frying
- 1 cup of self-rising flour
- Apple peeled and grated
- Banana, peeled and sliced

Directions

- Measure a cup of flour into a bowl and add milk of the same quantity to the bowl.
- Crack an egg into it. Whisk together until smooth.
- Place a large frying pan on a medium heat.
- Add a small knob of butter to melt.

- Add large spoonful of batter to the pan.
- Bake the pancake for 2 minutes and flip over, let bake for the same time.
- Wipe out the pan with a ball of kitchen paper, add another small knob of butter for the next batch.
- Serve and enjoy immediately.

Homemade candied peel

This recipe features great ingredients for a delicious taste typically lemons, oranges, and grapefruits.

Ingredients

- Rind of 1 grapefruit
- Rinds of 2 lemons
- 250g caster sugar
- Rinds of 2 oranges

Directions

- Add the fruit rinds to a large saucepan then cover with water.
- Bring to a boil.
- Lower the heat, let simmer and cook for 30 minutes.
- Drain excess water, let cool.
- Remove any remaining flesh from the peel and discard.
- In a medium saucepan, combine the caster sugar with 250ml of water, let simmer over a medium heat to dissolve the sugar, and the liquid is gently bubbling.

- Add the rinds, stir to combine.
- Lower the heat let simmer for 25 minutes.
- Remove from heat and leave to cool in the syrup.
- Preheat the oven to the lowest setting.
- Transfer the rinds to a wire rack set over a baking tray in the oven for 2 hours.
- Remove from the oven and toss in a little caster sugar.
- Serve and enjoy.

Archie's royal roulade

This is a fruity Mediterranean Sea diet desert featuring variety of fruity to provide you with your daily vitamin dose.

Ingredients

- 3 sprigs of fresh mint
- 7g of freeze-dried strawberries
- 200g of golden caster sugar
- 1 tablespoon of vanilla extract
- 1 tablespoon of icing sugar
- 1 lemon
- 400g of strawberries
- 150g of plain flour
- 6 large free-range eggs
- 150g of quality strawberry jam
- 3 tablespoons of elderflower cordial
- 1 vanilla pod
- 600ml of double cream

Directions

- Hull and finely slice 6 strawberries.
- Line a baking tray with greaseproof paper.

- Organize the strawberries in six evenly spaced rows across the tray.
- Place the tray in a cold oven and heat 350°F.
- Once the oven comes up to temperature, remove the tray of strawberries.
- Crack the eggs into a large mixing bowl.
- Add the sugar together with the vanilla extract, beat for 5 minutes.
- Grate the lemon zest, then sift and fold in the flour until smooth.
- Pour the mixture over the baked strawberries and smooth, bake for 15 minutes.
- Remove the sponge from the oven, peel off the original greaseproof paper.
- Place another sheet of greaseproof paper on your work-surface and scatter over 1 tablespoon of caster sugar.
- Flip the sponge back onto it.
- Chop the remaining strawberries, place in a bowl with the jam and elderflower cordial. Mix, let macerate.

- Halve the vanilla pod and scrape out the seeds into a clean mixing bowl.
- Add the cream and icing sugar, whisk.
- Transfer to a large piping bag with a nozzle.
- Grind the freeze-dried strawberries in a food processor to a dust.
- Unfold the cooled sponge, spread all over with the macerated strawberries and elderflower mixture.
- Pipe over most of the cream, gently roll the sponge back up.
- Trim the ends to neaten, and transfer to a serving board.
- Serve and enjoy.

Mixed leaf salad with mozzarella, mint, peach, and prosciutto

Ingredients

- Higher-welfare prosciutto
- Fresh mint
- Mixed salad leaves
- Lemon
- Ripe peach
- Extra virgin olive oil
- Dried red chilli
- Buffalo mozzarella

Directions

- Pinch the skin of the peaches.
- Peel from the bottom to the top, then divide into quarter.
- Rip the mozzarella into small pieces and place on a plate with the peaches.
- Season with sea salt and black pepper to taste.
- Lay a couple of slices of prosciutto over the top.
- Tear up the mint leaves, toss with the mixed salad leaves.

- Then, dress with a little of the extra virgin olive oil and lemon juice dressing.
- Place the leaves on top.
- Serve and enjoy.

Frozen fruit and almond crumble

This game has elevated making of a crumble to a whole new level with frozen fruit breaking the protocol of using dry fruits. In 45 minutes this recipe will be just ready.

Ingredients

- 100g of plain flour
- 1kg of mixed frozen berries and cherries
- 100g of flaked almonds
- ½ of an orange
- 50g of unsalted butter
- 100g of sugar

Directions

- Preheat your oven to 400°F.
- Place frozen berries into a saucepan with half the sugar.
- Place on a medium heat.
- Add in the juice of half an orange let cook for 8 minutes.
- Remove from the heat let cool briefly.
- Place butter in a mixing bowl with the flour.

- Rub together with your fingertips, then stir in the almonds and remaining sugar.
- Transfer the berry mixture to a baking dish.
- Sprinkle over the crumble topping.
- Let bake for 30 minutes.
- Serve and enjoy with vanilla ice cream.

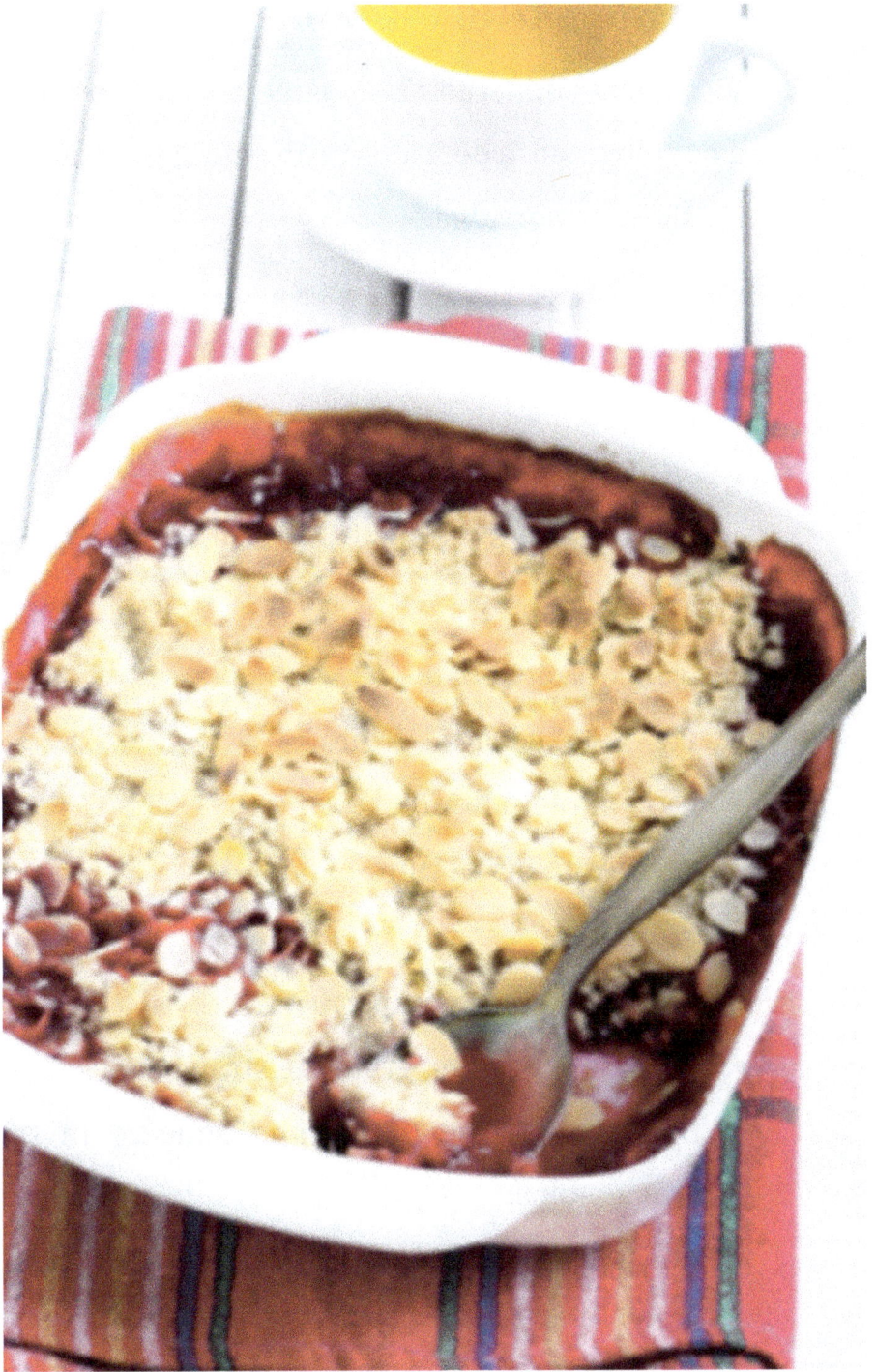

Roasted stone fruit crumble

Start by roasting your fruits then later, add the toppings to bring out the intense delicious taste with the incredible texture of the oats porridge.

Ingredients

- 8 strawberries
- 1 orange
- 50g of flaked almonds
- 75g of unsalted butter
- 75g of sugar
- 100g of rolled oats
- 1kg of mixed stone fruit
- 100g of plain flour
- 2 tablespoons of runny honey

Directions

- Preheat your oven to 400°F.
- Prepare the fruits, grate the strawberries.
- Drizzle over the honey and squeeze in the orange juice.
- Roast in the oven until the fruit is softened and juicy.

- Place butter in a mixing bowl with the flour.
- Rub together with your fingertips.
- Add the oats, almonds, and sugar.
- When cooked, sprinkle over the crumble topping.
- Then, return to the oven until golden and crunchy.
- Serve and enjoy with ice cream.

The quickest berry tart

This recipe finds it competitive advantage from its flavors together with the texture. For the berry lovers, trust me this recipe could not be any sweeter.

Ingredients

- 600g of mixed seasonal berries
- 1 splash of milk
- olive oil
- 1 orange
- 1 large free-range egg
- 3 tablespoons vanilla sugar
- 250g of plain flour
- 50g of icing sugar
- 4 meringue nests
- 125g of unsalted butter
- 400ml of double cream

Directions

- Sieve the flour and icing sugar into a large mixing bowl.

- Work butter cubes into the flour and sugar with your fingers until the mixture resembles breadcrumbs.
- Beat the egg, add to the mix with the milk and gently work it together with your hands until you have a ball.
- Sprinkle some flour over the dough and a clean work surface, and pat the ball into a thick flat round.
- Sprinkle over a little more flour, then wrap the pastry in Clingfilm.
- Refrigerate for 30 minutes.
- Serve and enjoy.

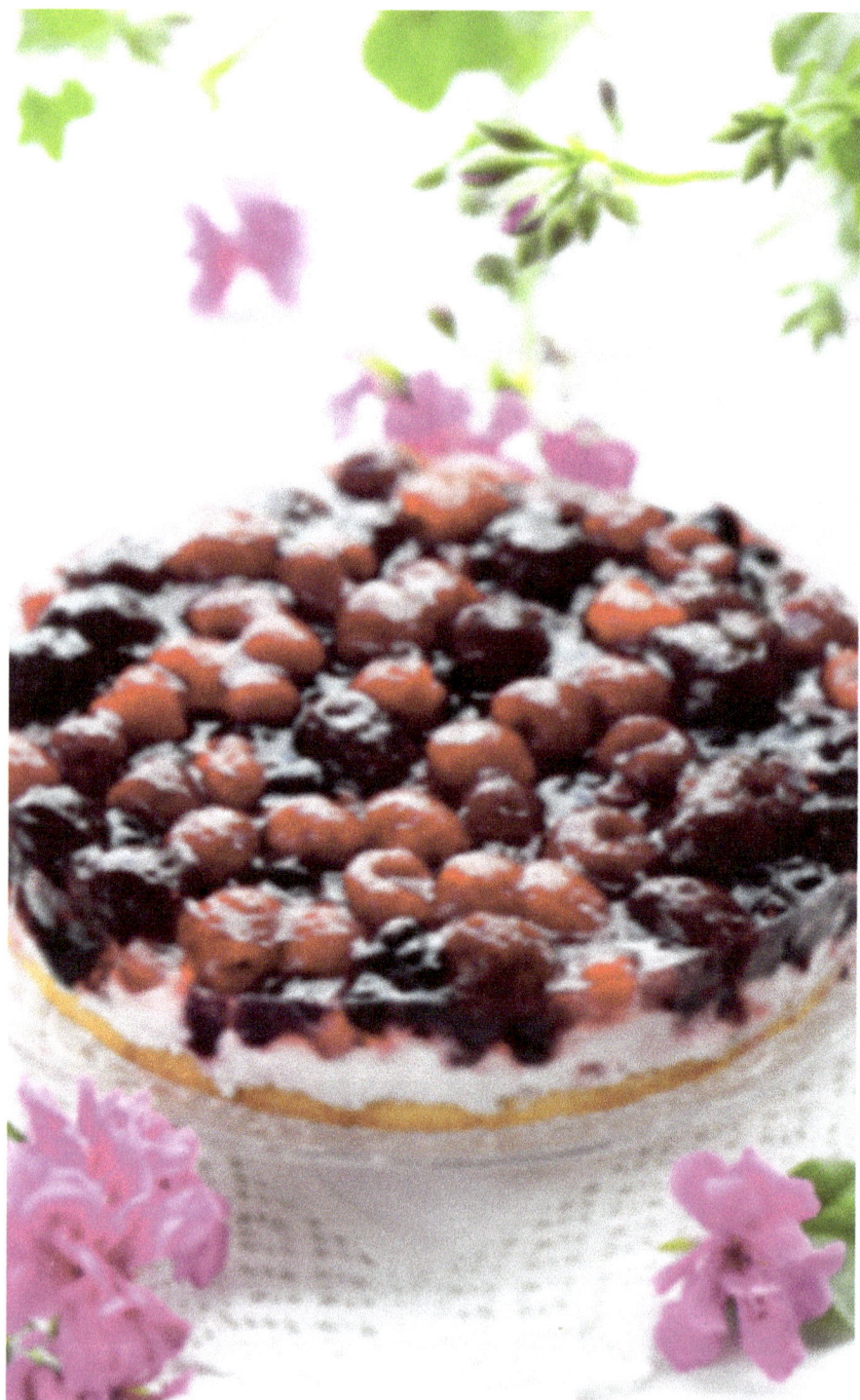

Tropical fruit pavlova

This recipe is the heart of the people in the southern hemisphere packed with variety of fruits, soft whipped cream, and irresistibly naturally sweet honey.

Ingredients

- 2 tamarillos
- 6 large free-range egg whites
- Runny honey
- 300g of caster sugar
- 8 passion fruits
- 1 teaspoon white wine vinegar
- ½ of a pineapple
- Oil
- 300ml of double cream
- 2 bananas

Directions

- Preheat the oven to 300°F.
- Grease and align a baking tray.
- Whisk the egg whites with a pinch of sea salt with an electric mixer, until soft peaks form.

- Add sugar, 1 tablespoon at a time until fully incorporated.
- Fold the vinegar into the meringue mix, then spoon onto the tray.
- Make a well in the center let bake for 1 hour.
- Turn off the oven when meringue is crisp, let cool down.
- Peel and slice the pineapple and bananas.
- Quarter the tamarillos.
- When the meringue is cooled, spread over the whipped cream and top with the cut fruit.
- Halve the passion fruits and scoop the pulp over the pavlova.
- Serve and enjoy.

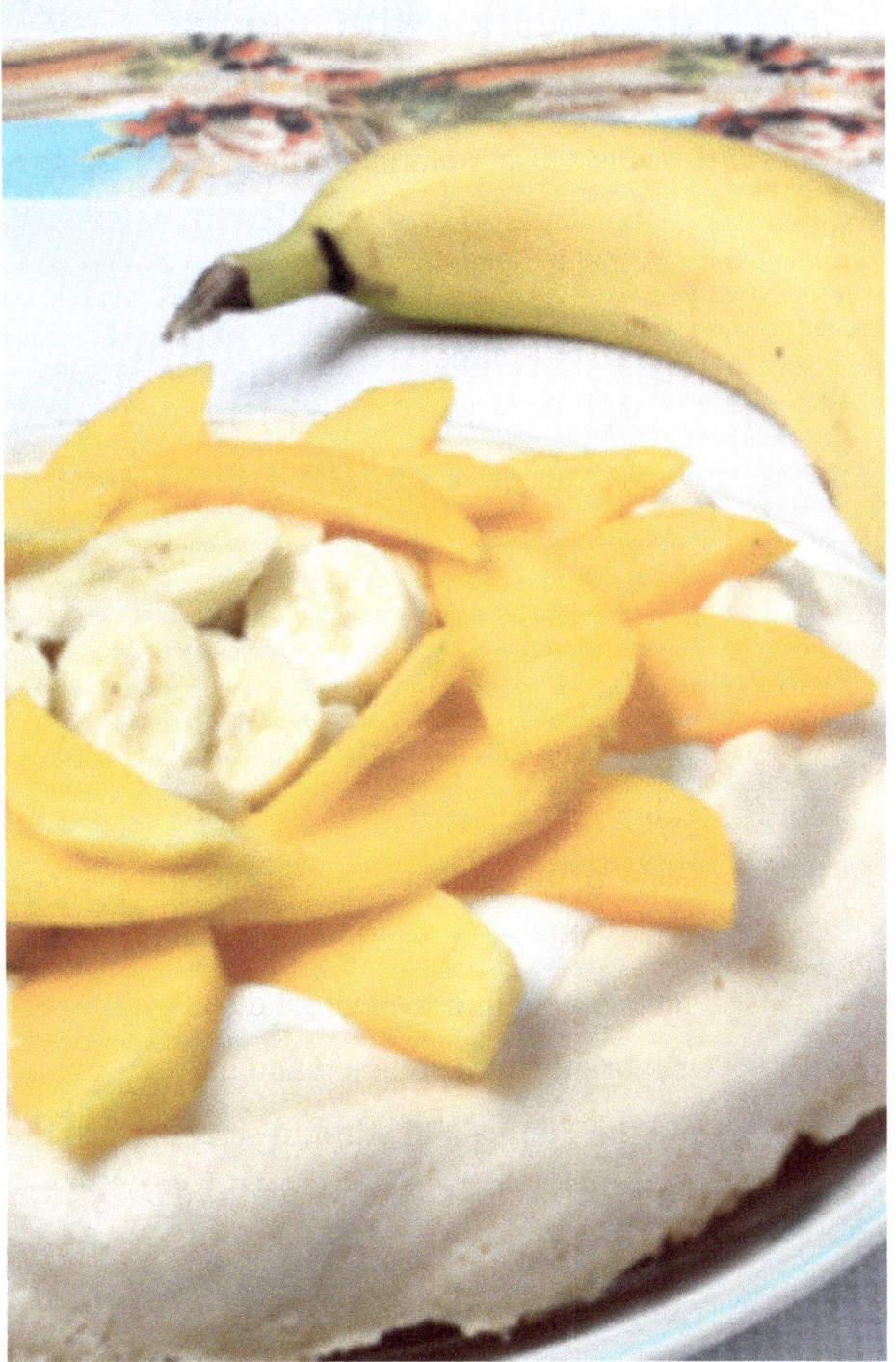

Grilled strawberries with pimms

Grilling a strawberry brings out a tasty flavor and they are iconic with no taste disappointments mainly with a ginger spice.

Ingredients

- 1 splash of Pimms
- 4 scoops of quality vanilla ice cream
- 1 tablespoon of vanilla sugar
- 1 tablespoon stem ginger
- 400g of strawberries

Directions

- Preheat the grill to high temperature.
- Hull the strawberries and toss with the sugar.
- Slice, stir the ginger through the strawberries with 2 tablespoons of the gingery syrup.
- Place in a shallow ovenproof dish.
- Grill briefly until softened and hot.
- Add the Pimms and stir and scrape up all the sticky bits from the bottom of the dish.
- Serve and enjoy.

Rolled cassata

This Mediterranean recipe originated from the Arabic influence desert with a silky smooth ricotta featuring nuts and chocolate. This recipe could not have been any better.

Ingredients

- 3 tablespoons of apricot jam
- 75g of plain flour
- 1 teaspoon of vanilla bean paste
- 100g of shelled unsalted pistachios
- 100g of quality dark chocolate
- 15 glacé of cherries
- 500g of white marzipan
- 3 large free-range eggs
- Icing sugar
- 50ml of vin Santo
- 400g of quality ricotta cheese
- 1 tablespoon caster sugar
- 50g of whole hazelnuts
- 100g of golden caster sugar
- 1 heaped tablespoon of glacé fruit
- Unsalted butter

- 20g of shelled unsalted pistachios

Directions

- Preheat the oven to 350°F.
- Whisk the eggs and sugar with an electric mixer.
- Sift in the flour, then add the vanilla paste and fold through.
- Grease a baking tray with butter.
- Spoon batter into the tray let bake for 15 minutes.
- Blend the pistachios in a food processor until fine.
- Break in the marzipan blend to form a dough
- Take the sponge out of the oven, Peel off the greaseproof.
- Place it back on top, and roll up while the sponge is still warm.
- Let cool for 20 minutes.
- In a food processor, whisk the ricotta with the sugar until smooth.
- Toast the hazelnuts until golden.

- Mix chopped glacé fruit, pistachios and chocolate into the ricotta.
- Roll out most of the marzipan on a large sheet of greaseproof paper.
- Spread over the jam, unroll the sponge on top.
- Drizzle over the Vin Santo and spread over the ricotta.
- Line up the cherries along the side, roll it up, pressing lightly to seal.
- Trim the ends, then roll out the remaining marzipan.
- Let chill in for 30 minutes.
- Serve and enjoy.

Watermelon granite

Ingredients

- 8 tablespoons of natural yoghurt
- 2 limes
- 1 small watermelon
- ½ of a bunch of fresh mint
- 60g of stem ginger in syrup

Directions

- Chop the watermelon flesh into chunks.
- Chop the ginger, place in a large freezer bag together with the watermelon chunks.
- Add the lime zest, freeze for 9 hours.
- Tip in the frozen watermelon mixture and blitz to a pink snow.
- Serve and enjoy.

Chocolate hot cross buns

The chocolate hot cross buns are elevated following this Mediterranean recipe with a massive delicious taste served warm.

Ingredients

- 150g quality dark chocolate
- 1 whole nutmeg
- 3 tablespoons of runny honey
- 50g of golden caster sugar
- Sachet of dried yeast
- 200ml of semi-skimmed milk
- 50g of unsalted butter
- 1 large free-range egg
- 400g of strong white bread flour
- 50g of quality cocoa powder
- 1 heaped teaspoon of mixed spice
- 100g of raisins or mixed dried fruit

Directions

- Combine butter, mixed spice, sugar, nutmeg, and a pinch of sea salt in a pan over a low heat, stirring occasionally until melted.

- Pour in milk, crack in the egg and whisk.
- Sift the flour and cocoa powder into a large bowl, add yeast.
- Make a well in the middle, pour in the milk mixture, form a rough dough.
- Transfer to a flour-dusted bowl, cover for 1 hour 30 minutes.
- When the dough is ready, transfer to a clean surface.
- Stretch and flatten the dough, sprinkle over the chocolate chips and dried fruit, knead until smooth.
- Preheat your oven to 350°F.
- Divide the dough into 12 equal pieces.
- Flatten one, push a piece of chocolate into the center, trap it inside.
- Repeat this with the remaining dough.
- Mix 2 tablespoons of flour with adequate water to a thick batter consistency, then transfer to a piping bag.
- Pipe thin crosses across the top of the buns.

- Let bake for 25 minutes, transfer to a cooling rack.
- Warm the honey, then gently brush over the buns to glaze.
- Serve and enjoy.

Pineapple carpaccio

Pineapples gifted to aid digestion and replace the vitamin deficiency, this recipe is a perfect choice to consume pineapple blended with blue berries.

Ingredients

- 1 lime
- 1 ripe pineapple
- 1 bunch of fresh mint
- 4 tablespoons of Greek-style coconut yoghurt
- 100g of blueberries

Directions

- Pick the mint leaves into mortar. Reserve some for later.
- Pound the rest into a paste, then muddle in 2 tablespoons of extra virgin olive oil.
- Top and tail the pineapple, then slice off the skin.
- Slice and arrange them on a large platter.
- Halve the blueberries, then sprinkle over the top.

- Ripple some mint oil through the yoghurt, spoon over the fruit.
- Grate over lime zest over the juice.
- Slice and sprinkle over the reserved mint leaves.
- Serve and enjoy.

Pineapples relish

Ingredients

- 1 lime
- 1 clove of garlic
- 3 fresh red chilies
- 2 tablespoons brown sugar
- 1 small ripe pineapple
- 2 fresh bird's-eye chilies
- 2 shallots

Directions

- Prepare the pineapples into wedges.
- Pulse the garlic and shallot in a food processor until fairly fine.
- Pulse in the pineapple until fine, but still with a texture.
- Stir in the sugar, pulse to combine.
- Squeeze and stir in the lime juice.
- Season to with sea salt and black pepper.
- Serve and enjoy.

Blackcurrant ombre cheesecake

Ingredients

- 4 sheets of gelatin
- 200g of blackcurrants and blackberries
- 1 vanilla pod
- 500g of light cream cheese
- 300ml of double cream
- 300g of oaty biscuits
- 100g of unsalted butter
- 340g of jars of Tiptree blackcurrant jam

Directions

- Oil the sides of a cake tin and line the base with greaseproof paper.
- In a large saucepan, melt the butter over a low heat.
- Blend the biscuits in a food processor until ground.
- Stir into the butter.
- Press the crumbs evenly into the tin, then leave in the fridge for 20 minutes.

- In a separate bowl, whisk the vanilla cream to soft peaks.
- Fold into the cream cheese with 1 heaped teaspoon of jam.
- Spoon a thick layer over the biscuit base.
- Add 1 heaped tablespoon of jam to the rest of the mixture, and another layer to the cheesecake.
- Soak the gelatin in cold water for 5 minutes, then drain.
- Spoon the remaining ½ jar of jam in a saucepan over a low heat with water and berries let simmer for 3 minutes.
- Stir in the gelatin until dissolved.
- Pour the jelly over the cheesecake, spread over the surface.
- Let it firm in the fridge for 1 hour.
- Serve and enjoy.

Christmas pudding

Ingredients

- 1 large free-range egg
- 150g of pecan nuts
- 75g of crystallized ginger
- 200ml of semi-skimmed milk
- 1 clementine
- Unsalted butter
- Barrel-aged bourbon
- 150g of Medjool dates
- 150g of dried apricots
- 1 small sprig of fresh rosemary
- 150g of dried cranberries
- 150g of raisins
- 150g of suet
- 150g of plain flour
- 75g of fresh breadcrumbs
- Golden syrup

Directions

- Oil a pudding bowl with butter.

- Combine the apricots, pecans, ginger and rosemary leaves in a food processor and blend.
- Place it all in a mixing bowl with the cranberries, raisins, suet, flour, breadcrumbs and milk.
- Break in the egg.
- Add clementine zest, squeeze in the juice and mix.
- Place bit of the mixture into the greased bowl and cover with a single layer of greaseproof paper and a double layer of tin foil.
- Tie a piece of string around the bowl to secure them in place and make it watertight.
- Let sit in a large, deep saucepan and pour in enough water to come halfway up the sides of the bowl.
- Boil, cover the pan with a tight-fitting lid.
- Lower the heat let simmer for 4 hours.
- Remove the foil and paper when time is up, turn out the pudding to a plate ready to serve.
- Enjoy.

Apple and date pie

A combination of apple and a pie is a favorite to most people spiced with dates and cinnamon.

Ingredients

- 1 large free-range egg
- 140g of unsalted butter
- 275g of plain flour
- 1 teaspoon of milk
- 1 tablespoon of demerara sugar
- 3 bramley apples
- 6 brae burn apples
- 5 Medrol dates
- 4 tablespoons of soft light muscovite sugar
- ¼ teaspoon of ground cinnamon
- 1 lemon
- 1 large free-range egg yolk
- 1 pinch of ground cloves

Directions

- Place diced butter and flour in a food processor as well as teaspoon of sea salt, then pulse until the coarse.

- Squeeze in 1 tablespoon of lemon juice.
- Add the egg yolk with 2 tablespoons of cold water, blend to combine.
- Divide the dough in two, let chill in the fridge for 1 hour.
- Place in core apples in a saucepan.
- Sprinkle over the reserved lemon zest and squeeze in the remaining juice.
- Stir in the dates with the sugar and spices.
- Let simmer for 8 minutes over a medium-low. Set aside to cool.
- Preheat the oven to 400°F.
- Roll one of the pastry discs out to 5mm thick on a clean, floured surface and use it to line a deep 20cm pie dish, pushing the pastry into the edges.
- Spoon in the cooled pie filling.
- Roll the second pastry disc out to 5mm thick, brush the edges with water and place over the pie, pressing the edges to seal.
- Fold in the overhang and crimp with your fingers.

- Combine free range eggs, milk, and demerara in a small bowl, brush all over the pie.
- Make incisions into the pie top.
- Sprinkle with extra demerara sugar.
- Let bake for 40 minutes.
- Serve and enjoy.

Sticky cinnamon fog and yogurt breakfast bowls

This recipe makes a perfect start for a person's weekday or weekend with the crunchy granola or creamy yogurt.

Ingredients

- 600g of Greek yoghurt
- ¼ teaspoon of cinnamon
- 2 tablespoons of unsalted pistachio nuts
- 4 tablespoons of fresh unsweetened orange juice
- 4 tablespoons of granola
- 4 tablespoons of runny honey
- 150g of blackberries
- 8 ripe figs

Directions

- Preheat your oven to 400°F.
- Halve the figs and arrange cut-side up on a lined baking tray.
- In a small bowl, whisk the cinnamon together with the orange juice and honey until combined, then spoon over the figs.

- Let roast for 15 minutes, or until tender and sticky.
- Scatter the blackberries over the figs and return to the oven for 3 minutes.
- Top with the roasted fruit, reserving the juices in the tray.
- Scatter the granola and pistachios over the pots and drizzle with the reserved juices.
- Serve and enjoy.

Oat, pear and cardamom smoothie

Ingredients

- 2 teaspoons of bee pollen
- 500ml of oat milk
- 2 teaspoons of runny honey
- 2 pears
- 6 cardamom pods
- 100g of natural yoghurt

Directions

- Prepare the pears a night prior.
- Open the cardamom pods and extract the seeds, then crush up in a pestle.
- Place the crushed seeds into a blender.
- Add the frozen pears together with the oat milk, yoghurt, and honey, blend till smooth.
- Serve and sprinkle with bee pollen.
- Enjoy.

Aperol and grapefruit citrus jellies

Ingredients

- 4 grapefruits
- 50g of caster sugar
- 100ml of double cream
- 1 teaspoon of icing sugar
- 1 lemon
- 1 orange
- 75ml of Aperol
- 8 leaves of gelatin

Directions

- Soak the gelatin in cold water for 5 minutes.
- Cut the zested fruits in half and squeeze the juice into a pan.
- Add water together with the Aperol, sugar, and soaked gelatin.
- Heat gently until the gelatin and sugar have dissolved. Let cool.
- Place the remaining grapefruit into the jelly mix.

- Pour into 8 clean glasses refrigerate for 3 hours.
- Pour the cream over the citrus zest and add the icing sugar.
- Beat until soft peaks form and then spoon on top of the set jellies.
- Serve and enjoy.

Pineapple pancake mess

This recipe utilizes over ripened and sweeter pineapple with abundant manganese minerals to boost metabolism of the body. The recipe features cinnamon as a flavor and vanilla extract.

Ingredients

- 2 tablespoons of unsweetened desiccated coconut flakes
- 1 ripe pineapple
- Manuka honey
- 1 large free-range egg
- olive oil
- 4 tablespoons of natural yoghurt
- 4 cardamom pods
- 150g of plain whole meal flour
- 1 lime
- 300ml of semi-skimmed milk
- 1 teaspoon of vanilla extract
- 1 pinch of ground cinnamon
- 40g cashew nuts

Directions

- Toast the cashews.
- Add the coconut for briefly.
- Place both into a pestle, lightly crush.
- Return the dry pan to a medium-high heat, cook the pineapple for 10 minutes, place on a warm plate.
- Place the cardamom seeds into a blender with the flour, vanilla extract, milk, egg, cinnamon, and a tiny pinch of sea salt. Blend until smooth.
- Drizzle with small oil into the empty pineapple pan.
- Wipe it around.
- Add enough batter to lightly cover the base of the pan.
- Let cook until golden on both sides, then remove to a second plate.
- Repeat the process, stacking up the pancakes, covering with a tea towel.
- Serve and enjoy.

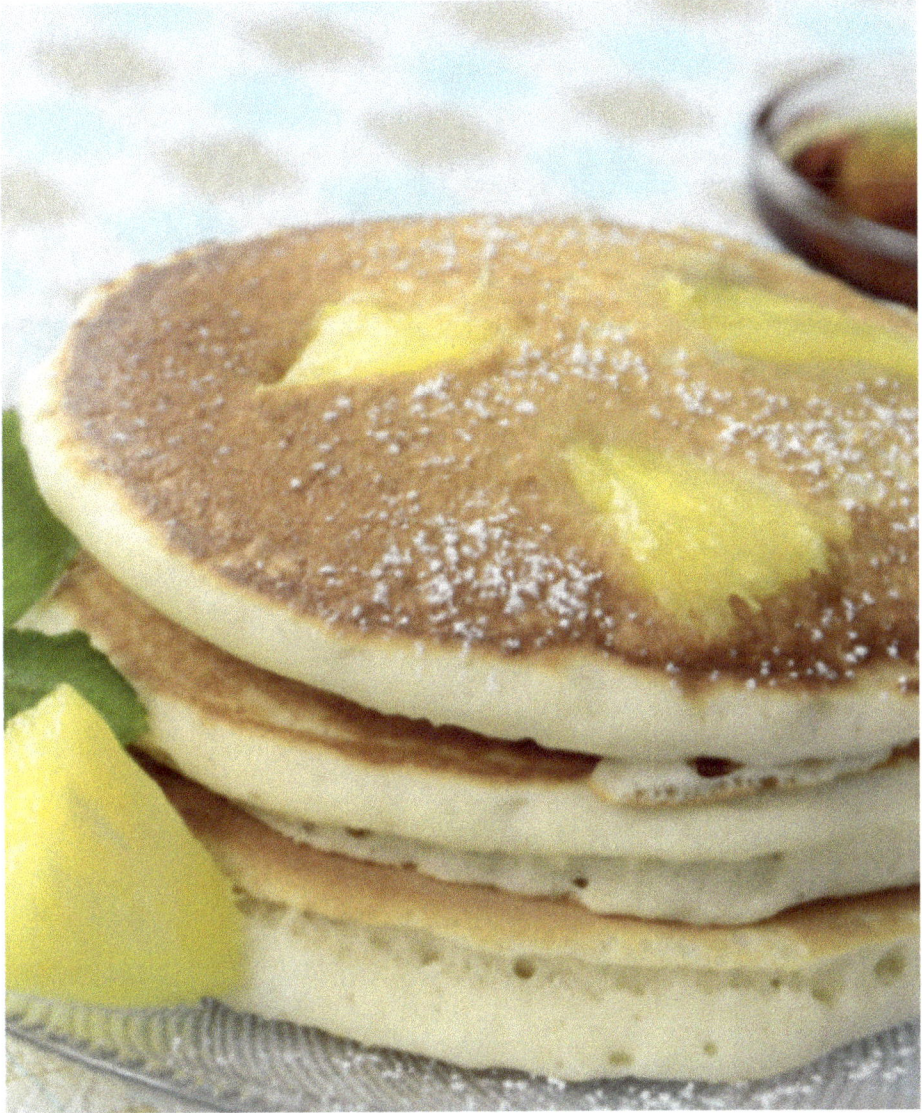

www.ingramcontent.com/pod-product-compliance
Lightning Source LLC
Chambersburg PA
CBHW062119040426
42336CB00041B/1932